Carolyn's Journey

David
Love
Grandma
Carol
& Grandpa
Victor
Anderson

CAROLYN'S JOURNEY

From Parkinson's Disease To A Nearly Normal Life
After Deep Brain Stimulation

By Victor Anderson

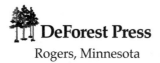

DeForest Press
Rogers, Minnesota

Notice: This book is intended as a reference guide, not as a medical manual, and the information is intended to help you make informed decisions about your health. It is not a substitute for treatment recommended to you by your doctor.

Permission gratefully acknowledged for the following:
    The drawing of Jesus by Derek Lusche on page 69.
    Use of the mnemonic for Parkinson disease patients considering Deep Brain Stimulation by Dr. Michael Okun, MD and Dr. KellyFoote, MD on page 54.

Published by:
DeForest Press
P.O. Box 383
Rogers, MN 55374 USA
www.DeForestPress.com
Toll-free: 866-509-0604
Richard DeForest Erickson, Founder
Shane Groth, Publisher

Cover design by Linda Walters, Optima Graphics, Appleton, WI

ISBN 1-930374-23-2
Printed in the United States of America
09 08 07 06   5 4 3 2 1

                Library of Congress Cataloging-in-Publication Data

Anderson, Victor (Carl Victor)
 Carolyn's journey : from Parkinson disease to a nearly normal life after deep brain stimulation / by Victor Anderson.
   p. cm.
 ISBN 1-930374-23-2
   1. Anderson, Carolyn, 1944---Health. 2. Parkinson's disease--Patients--Biography. I. Title.
 RC382.A62 2006
 362.196'8330092--dc22
 [B]
         2006011767

This book is dedicated to our parents,
Mr. and Mrs. Allen and Irene Bedsted,
and Ruth T. and Carl Victor Anderson Sr.

About the Quilts

The different quilts appearing at the beginning of each chapter were made by Carolyn during her past twenty years living with Parkinson's disease. They are also symbolic of the random pieces of information people with Parkinson's must deal with on a daily basis and how, through help, the pieces can begin to come together to form a pattern of normalcy.

Contents

Preface

This book follows the journey of Carolyn Anderson, my wife, over the nearly twenty years while she struggled with Parkinson's disease. She lived the first seven years with her disease without knowing what was wrong with her. I felt it was important to share some of our experiences so that readers could learn what to expect if they are diagnosed with Parkinson's. While I've tried to cover the symptoms that directly affected Carolyn, I've also attempted to explain some of the symptoms that were never an issue with her. Still, there is no way that all of the variations or symptoms of Parkinson's disease can be included in this book. I've also included how a person's life can change if they elect to have Deep Brain Stimulation surgery (DBS), as well as how Activa® Therapy may lead them back to a nearly normal life.

Just a warning. We tell both the good parts of the story as well as the places where the going got tough

Activa® and Activa® Therapy are registered trademarks of Medtronic, Inc.

and how those times impacted the decision-making process that Carolyn went though. Some of the decisions that involved the actual surgery itself may bring a tear to your eye, others may make you smile. Because we're already giving away the fact that Carolyn is here and much better for the journey, you'll realize that the outcome was a good one and that nothing good ever comes without some sacrifice.

This is a story as much about the spiritual blessings in one's life as it is about the disease and the therapy. In Carolyn's case, the blessings that have come with the decision to have the surgery are such that she would never go back to life without the assistance of Activa Therapy. In spite of the problems and complications experienced along the journey, it has all been worth it in the long run for the chance of living a nearly normal life.

Our first hint that something was wrong started in the 1980s and we will bring you, the reader, up to date through the surgery and the implementation of the Activa Therapy.

Carolyn and I wish to thank the following doctors who have supported her through diagnosis, disability retirement, and DBS surgery and follow-up: Steven Stein, Shelly Svoboda, M. Sullivan, Paul Tuite, and surgeon Robert Maxwell. Also special thanks to Carolyn's nurse, Maggie Bebler, and Drs. Okun and Foote at the University of Florida, Gainesville.

Introduction

Parkinson's disease is a chronic, progressively degenerating brain disorder of the nervous system. It affects a person's motor controls and is the direct result of a significant reduction of nerve cells called the substantia nigra die, or more commonly known as the "black substance". These nerve cells produce a chemical called "dopamine". Dopamine is the chemical messenger that transmits signals within the brain that control the body's muscles allowing for smooth and coordinated movement. In Parkinson's, the loss of the nerve cells results in decreased levels of dopamine causing interrupted signals to the brain. Therefore muscle movement is less smooth and uncoordinated. Dopamine can be replaced by medications, but the dosage needs to be increased over time to produce the same results. Eventually the dosage needed becomes too high for patients to tolerate without experiencing severe side affects and the affects of the disease become acutely debilitating.

Parkinson's disease is named after an English doctor named James Parkinson who described the condition in 1817. He did such a thorough study that today's researchers and clinicians are still urged to read his original notes on the condition.

The signs and symptoms of Parkinson's, which often appear gradually yet with increasing severity, may include tremors or trembling (uncontrolled shaking usually affecting one side of the patient more than the other); difficulty maintaining balance and gait; rigidity or stiffness of the limbs, face and trunk (called dyskensia); and general slowness of movement (also called bradykinesia). Patients may also eventually have difficulty walking, talking, or completing other simple tasks. Other signs include the patient's handwriting becoming smaller and cramped, uncontrolled facial movement, a shuffling walk, muffled speech and depression.

While Carolyn did not suffer from all of these symptoms, her numerous falls (including the one that broke her ankle), the muscle cramping (particularly while riding in the car), as well as the tremors (an almost constant condition) and the duskiness of her facial appearance were textbook examples of these symptoms.

What causes the condition and who gets it? The exact cause is not known, but most believe it is a combination of genetic and environmental factors. No definitive data exists. Onset usually occurs later in life, usually past the age of fifty, although some cases have involved people under the age of thirty. Each year, approximately 60,000 people are diagnosed with Parkinson's.

Most patients are Caucasians, with more men than women being affected. There is a strange connection to the northern European and Scandinavian countries. Over the years, a large number of immigrants from those regions have settled in the five-state area around Minnesota. Today that five-state area has the highest concentration of Parkinson's patients in America with North Dakota having the greatest percentage.

Deep Brain Stimulation (DBS) is an FDA-approved surgical treatment for Parkinson's disease. It is not a cure. Activa Therapy (by Medtronic, Inc.) uses neurostimulator(s) implanted near the collar, sometimes called a "brain pacemaker", to power electrodes implanted in the brain to stimulate the brain cells to send signals to the body's muscles for smooth and coordinated movement. These signals mimic the way dopamine works in people who have not had a reduction of nerve cells as a result of Parkinson's. With Activa Therapy, the patient can, in many situations, improve his or her ON time. You will hear the term ON time occasionally throughout this story. It refers to the best of conditions while on medication. If the patient still experiences symptoms while on his or her medication, or if the medication seems to quit or not last until the time for the next scheduled dose, the patient's ON time is decreased. OFF time is the period when the patient does not receive relief from the symptoms of Parkinson's disease despite having taken medication.

Introduction

For Carolyn, her ON time increased significantly after the surgery.

DBS is a major advance in the treatment of Parkinson's disease, The more neurosurgeons that become involved in this area of controlling the debilitating effects of Parkinson's, the more the knowledge base grows and implantation techniques will be improved all to the patient's benefit. There are two areas of the brain that are commonly the targets of stimulation. An MRI helps map the brain for placement of the electrodes. While communicating with the patient, the doctors can see the immediate results at the time of the surgery.

A temporary device is installed on the patient's head before the surgery begins. The purpose of the device is to hold the patient's head in place during surgery so that the doctors can make sure the DBS electrodes are inserted correctly into the brain to produce the desired results.

According to the National Parkinson Foundation website, there is a new case of Parkinson's diagnosed every nine minutes (see www.parkinson.org for more information). You may also want to check out the following, which we found extremely helpful: Michael J. Fox's Foundation at www.michealjfox.org/parkinsons, and the American Parkinson Disease Association at www.apdaparkinson.org. For more information about the Activa Therapy you may visit the Medtronic website at www.medtronic.com/parkinsons/activa or www.newhopeforparkinsons.com.

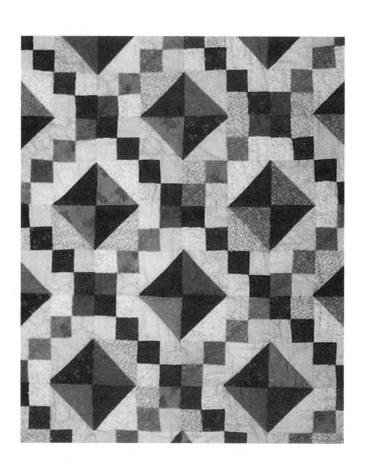

1

Chapter One

In the Beginning

We were staying in bed late one Saturday morning and watching TV. Our home had a large bedroom suite complete with a walk-in closet and adjacent master bath. Carolyn got up to go to the bathroom; when she got out of bed she promptly fell flat on her face in a bunch of blankets lying on her side of the bed. At first I was shocked. I jumped up and made sure she was alright. When I realized that she was OK, we laughed about it. She picked herself up

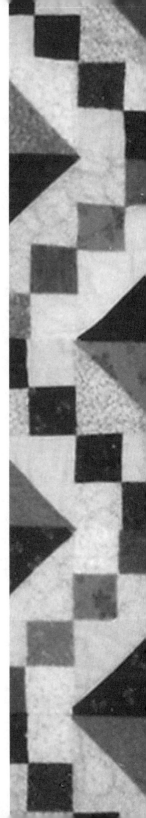

and continued to the bathroom. This was around the summer of 1988 and was one of the earliest symptoms of Parkinson's for Carolyn.

Part of the reason we took this first incident so lightly was our lack of knowledge about Parkinson's at this time. The other reason is that we didn't think much about it until a couple of years later when we learned enough to understand what potentially happened that morning. We also didn't think anything like Parkinson's would happen to either of us.

Let me paint you a picture of our life at this time. I was employed at a major defense manufacture about a thirty-five mile commute from our home. Our home was in the little town of Zimmerman, Minnesota. The house was newly constructed next to Carolyn's parent's retirement home and was located on the beautiful shores of Lake Fremont (the largest lake in Sherburne County). It became a popular gathering spot for our already grown children and growing number of grandchildren. The house was everything we had dreamed of. It had three bedrooms, a split foyer, a lower level that was finished, a large master bedroom suite, a three-season porch and two-car garage. Lakeside we had made a beach and brought in some fine sand for our grandchildren to play in, as the lake itself has a muddy bottom, typical of a shallow lake. The yard was landscaped and the flowers were one of Carolyn's joys.

Carolyn is the "perfect daughter" and wanted to be there, right next door to her parents in their declining years. Both of my parents were gone and I sort of adopted them as surrogate parents for myself as well. Carolyn's dad had acted as on-sight quality control as the men worked on building our house. We were very close and seldom had any conflicts.

Carolyn worked at an electronic manufacturing company about four or five miles closer than my job, so we were able to commute together. I would drop her off at work and continue on to my job. Being able to commute together was great for our communications and Carolyn did not have to drive. This quality time together was precious to us. By March 1989 my work at the defense plant came to an end. So, consequently, our commuting days together also came to an end. But I digress.

Carolyn was active, kept up the house, and dabbled in oil painting as her way of relaxing. She also enjoyed other crafts, along with gardening, and became interested in quilting. We both enjoyed taking her folks' on pontoon boat for rides around the lake at sunset. I enjoyed golfing in Princeton, Minnesota. We all started attending the United Methodist Church in Princeton. You could say that back in those days we were a very typical mid-America family.

You might even say that at this time we were living the American dream. We had our dream house, next door to Carolyn's folks. We had designed the house so the master bedroom suite was our oasis when we were done with work and the commute home. (There is a reason they call these communities this far from town "bedroom communities.") There was a beautiful fireplace, done in granite so that it looked like the stone from nearby St. Cloud, Minnesota. The kitchen was also a source of pride as it was equipped with a built-in Jenn-Aire grill and all of the other major appliances that you would expect, plus an adjacent dining area. The yard was full of flowers that Carolyn loved to plant, care for, and watch grow. And being on the lakeshore demonstrated to us every day how blessed we were.

All of this background information may seem a bit trivial, but you'll soon see how most all of it would have bearing on Carolyn's journey.

Over the next few years, during the late 1980s and the early part of the 1990s, Carolyn's symptoms persisted and became more noticeable, with the tremor and the muscle cramping being the worst. Carolyn began thinking that these symptoms were related and there was something wrong with her. As the factors that affected her daily performance at work became more noticeable, they also began to have a bigger impact on her life. We had no idea what the cause was; she already started to have a slight tremor in her left arm and leg. When she rode in the car or just lounged around the house she could feel the muscles cramping, in her leg specifically, but also in her arm. She thought that perhaps she should talk to her doctor.

You might say that in the early '90s Carolyn's life started to fall apart. In early 1991 her mother had a heart attack. While in the hospital her mother suffered another attack that would take her life. Six weeks later we returned home from work to find that her dad had suffered a stroke. A couple of weeks later he too left this world for the Promised Land.

The dream house was starting to take its toll on Carolyn as well. Since it was a split-level, the stairs were involved in nearly every move. It was half a flight to get to the foyer from the main floor, another half flight to the lower level, and at least a couple steps down to the garage level. To go out the front door there were a couple of more steps down to the driveway. Out the back, toward the beach and the dock, there was a whole flight of stairs from the three-season porch. Climbing or walking down the stairs seemed to leave her with a lack of energy with every move she made, almost as though the stairs were zapping her energy. She was tempted to blame this lack of energy on the grieving process, or maybe depression, but other than the lack of energy she didn't think she was depressed. She thought, "I have a wonderful husband, great kids that are healthy, and grandchildren that are a blessing. I like my job, and in spite of everything else, I am very good at it. What more could I want?"

When it came time for her annual exam, Carolyn talked to a doctor—not her regular doctor—one doing the physical for the carpal tunnel problem she was experiencing at work. She thought she would make double use of this physical in order to avoid the delays involved in getting into our regular clinic.

During the consultation the doctor gave her a list of possibilities that could be associated with the symptoms Carolyn had mentioned. This short list of possible causes included Parkinson's disease, and because she included those things in her report, it was available for the disability insurance company to see during their investigation. We had no idea at the time the significant ramifications of what we thought was an innocent conversation.

We would learn that soon enough, and as a public service I include this in the hope of preventing a similar incident from occurring in your own personal journey. The short list that was discussed that day was later used by the disability insurance company to define the date of diagnosis for Carolyn's Parkinson's disease. Looking back now, after being around Parkinson's, we know that a true diagnosis takes neurologists much more than a lucky guess. The fact still remains that the insurance company used this doctor's "guess" to define the date of diagnosis, and in so doing had us between a rock and a hard place. We found ourselves without the ability to fight them. We thought they were trying to help us, and we had to accept this date of diagnosis as part of the ground rules. This would cost Carolyn thousands of dollars over the years. Because of the "diagnosis" at this time, the insurer canceled a ten percent increase that Carolyn had elected the next renewal date after this appointment. They also returned the premiums we had paid and prevented us from receiving the higher payout. That cost us dearly.

In defense of the insurance company, they did go to bat for Carolyn when they asked her employer for information about her work hours in order to calculate the disability amount she was eligible to receive. Before this time, the company's human resource manager had sent a letter to everyone in the company during one of its slower periods, telling employees they could sign up to work a reduced thirty-two hour work week. Carolyn thought this sounded very good as she wanted more time for her crafts and artwork. So, she signed up.

Although this would have been a very nice option, the company never allowed her or anyone else in her department to work thirty-two hours a week. Instead, she kept working the full forty hours. The company seemed to feel this was irrelevant when reporting to the insurance company, however, and claimed she worked thirty-two hours a week. Carolyn went to the payroll department and asked for a printout of her hours. The total came to an average of forty-two hours a week. Once we forwarded this information to the insurance company, they were really upset. When they discovered Carolyn's employer had never honored the thirty-two hour work week request and saw what the actual average hours worked were, they sent a strongly-worded letter back to the human resource manager saying that if she ever did that again there would be dire consequences. Carolyn received a part of the money lost by that bad diagnosis date decision by getting the company to own up to the actual number of hours she worked, including her overtime. We have always felt that she had been entitled to both.

Eventually Carolyn was referred to the Minneapolis Clinic of Neurology. This turned out to be the start of the actual diagnosis of Parkinson's disease. The doctor Carolyn was assigned to was extremely intelligent and always concerned for her patient's welfare. Carolyn's first appointment was on June 13, 1995.

(Just a sidebar here. Carolyn's birthday is the thirteenth. She has always been afraid of that day if her birthday fell on a Friday. She would be better off staying in bed as to get up at all).

The doctor examined Carolyn and ordered a number of tests. She discovered that Carolyn had the following symptoms and estimated that she had them for the last couple of years: 1) Intermittent cramping in her toes; 2) Stiffness in her fingers, preventing her from being efficient at work; and 3) Numbness in both legs if she sat for prolonged periods of time. In addition, for the last couple of months, she had experienced yet another associated symptom, intermittent gait imbalance. She also had been told by her friends that she was shaking in both hands while she herself had not noticed it. This is almost always true at first of Parkinson's disease patients.

Her doctor also questioned her about her past medical history, the medications Carolyn was taking, her social and family history, a list of her job duties, the fact that both parents were deceased and that Carolyn was a non-smoker. At this time there were no dystonic movements (the erratic facial movements) or wresting tremor (involuntary shaking of the arm or legs) during the examination. The doctor ordered a number of tests, as well as the results of previous tests conducted by Carolyn's primary care physician.

At Carolyn's next appointment on July 5, 1995, the doctor was calling the observed condition "Parkinsonian." And in less than a month Carolyn was demonstrating more Parkinson's symptoms. The doctor again ordered more tests, and by the third appointment was using "Parkinsonism" as her impression of the cause of Carolyn's symptoms.

Another area of concern for Carolyn at this appointment was that her breast implant might be the source of the problems she was experiencing. If the implant was leaking silicone into her body, might this be the cause of her symptoms? The doctor never acknowledged that it was or could have been the source contributing to her Parkinsonian symptoms.

Carolyn set up an appointment with the doctors that had originally put the silicone implant in after her mastectomy. They agreed that it would be best if the implant came out. So Carolyn went in and had the implant removed. The good news was that the implant had not developed any cracks nor had it began to leak silicone into her body. However, as they were removing the implant, the hardened silicone skin of the implant cracked and fell apart right after they had removed it from her chest. Carolyn always looked back on this as being a kind of divine intervention. Removing the implant may have avoided serious problems down the road.

After about six months the doctor concluded that Parkinson's was the correct diagnosis. The test, the motor skills, and the symptoms all added up. To make absolutely sure, however, the doctor recommended that Carolyn see another doctor at the Mayo Clinic in Rochester, Minnesota.

Our insurance provider approved this second opinion. I took a couple of days off work, and we struck out on a Friday morning for Rochester.

As we waited in the lobby outside the neurology clinic offices, Carolyn, nervous about the appointment, began counting the doctors' names on the wall. When she had reached about ninety, which was only a fraction of the names listed, the receptionist called her.

The doctor was a pleasant woman about forty and was very professional. She watched Carolyn walk back and forth across her office. She asked about the tremor and muscle cramping. Then, when Carolyn was standing in front of her, she grabbed her shoulders and pushed her backwards. Carolyn couldn't react fast enough, which was enough to indicate that Parkinson's disease was indeed the correct diagnosis. (By the way, this is the date we felt the insurance company should have considered the actual date of diagnosis.)

While we found our way back to the car we passed the Mayo Clinic bookstore and looked for a book or two that would shed some light on Parkinson's. Carolyn, after thinking for a moment, said, "I had heard that my dad's Aunt Hilda was in a nursing home in Wisconsin with Parkinson's. I also remember my dad shaking occasionally. At the time I didn't think much about anything being wrong with him. He never went to the doctor, but in looking back, he may have had the onset of Parkinson's. If he hadn't had the stroke, and the cigarettes hadn't shortened his life… But this is all 20/20 hindsight, and I really don't know if he had it or not. I guess we'll never know for sure. My life was so busy and we were so young and innocent, we never took time to think about anything like that happening to our parents."

We returned to our car and headed north toward home. I wasn't sure that I knew what to do or say at this point, but I tried to keep Carolyn's' spirits up on the way home. Let me say this. We did make a pact vowing that we would keep up our normal lifestyle as long as we could. We would not let this disease rule our life. We still took vacations and short day trips and still enjoy visiting or entertaining friends and family whenever possible. That day, as a matter of fact, we stopped at an outlet shopping center, as well as a local casino for some gaming and supper.

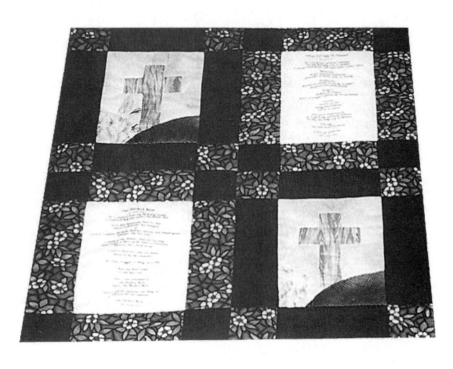

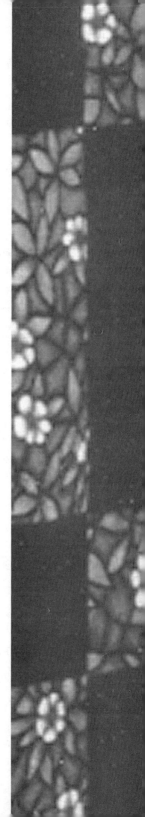

2

Chapter Two

Why Me, Lord?

Why me, Lord? Carolyn's answer from above didn't come easily, but while she wondered about this question, life went on.

At the time of diagnosis Carolyn had taken about a month off work. Carolyn had many more questions than she had answers. How fast does this progress? Can I keep working? How long? What about how I live my life away from work?

Our faith had brought us through this far and we were sure it would take us through whatever was to come. Carolyn really did believe that God would provide. She was sent to another doctor at the Minneapolis Clinic of Neurology, Dr. Steven Stein. The month off work helped her adjust to the first round of drugs, and by the end of the month she was feeling better, so she returned to work.

Dr. Stein prescribed the first round of medication and put her on Sine-met 25/100. This is the brand name of the drug Carbadopa/Levodopa and the 25/100 is the milligram content of each. Starting with only a couple pills a day at first, within a short time she was increased to four tablets per day, and she saw only minimal improvement. She still suffered from stiffness in her arm and hands and a tremor in her upper body.

These conditions were becoming more apparent and affected her ability to do her job. The assembly of the electronic sensors where she was employed took dexterity. Her work also included welding the leads onto the assembly, taking again another set of skills. Carolyn was not the first person to suffer from Parkinson's disease who also did welding, which made us wonder about a connection between the two. There is nothing official about welders getting Parkinson's; it's just an observation on our part.

The doctors at this time were monitoring Carolyn's copper levels as well as having her collect urine specimens. Everybody at this point seemed sure that Parkinson's disease was what Carolyn was suffering from and that her medication appeared to delay progression of the symptoms. Carolyn and I had great respect for Dr. Steven Stein, her primary Parkinson's doctor. I would often say that he was the Parkinson god of Minnesota.

As her medicine was increased, she found that her legs were still not working well. The tremor and muscle cramps were returning more quickly after medication, so her muscle control was maintained by increasing the amount and mix of drugs. Dr. Stein told her to continue working as long as he could. After that, Carolyn would apply for social security disability.

It was in the fall of 1996 when we sold the house on the lake. We had two reasons for changing our residence. The taxes on lakeshore property were going out of sight and the stairs were getting harder for Carolyn to manage. We went house hunting and purchased a three bedroom rambler on a nine-hole executive golf course about four miles from our present lake home. We gained lower taxes, lower payments, no stairs to climb, and a golf course. What more could we ask for?

One day on the way to work (Carolyn still commuted thirty miles to work daily), she got pulled over for speeding by a Minnesota state trooper. He let her go with just a warning, but it shook her up and she was quite nervous about driving after that. She didn't like driving all that well anyway, and the muscle cramping while driving added to the stress of the daily commute.

Carolyn didn't like it, but she continued to commute to work daily for about two more years. One day, around mid-October 1998, she was called into her supervisor's office and told that she should go home and not return until she was back physically at one hundred percent. Carolyn thought at first that her boss was joking, but he was dead serious. It was obvious he had no clue about what it meant to have Parkinson's disease.

Carolyn knew that she would never be able to do her job at one hundred percent again. She just packed up the pictures and her personal items from her workstation and walked out the door. She thought, "Is this how it ends? Is this all the thanks I get for giving them twenty-three years of my life? I feel hurt, like I'm a second class citizen. Not only have I worked here for twenty-three years, but two of my children also have worked here for fifteen years each. This whole situation is starting to gall me to no end. I think about seeing a lawyer. Then again, if I sue them, in the end they will just take it out on the kids."

In retrospect, it seemed odd that such an attitude existed in this company, especially since the person who started it and was still running everyday operations was also a victim of Parkinson's. When Carolyn got home she called the social security people and started the application process for her disability.

We called a lawyer and arranged a meeting. The attorney advised us that the best he could do was to monitor the proceedings and make sure Carolyn got all that she had coming. The disability insurer also was watching out for Carolyn's interests as they would benefit from a lower payout if she got everything that she had coming.

Later we set up an appointment with Dr. Stein, who requested that Carolyn send him the medical records from her social security documentation. He said he would take care of the rest. We didn't know what he meant at that time.

Our disability insurance company became involved at this point. This is where we had a controversy regarding the date of diagnosis. The disability insurance carrier told us they would supplement her income until social security payments began. The insurance company paid her the first month of disability pay because the Social Security Administration withheld her first payment. The insurance company told us we could pay them back when social security kicked in. They indicated social security would send her back pay starting the date the company had sent her home, minus one month.

Time moves slowly when you have all day to think about what is or is not happening. Carolyn felt out of control, or so it seemed. To her, it seemed that the rest of the world was controlling her life and she really didn't have a say in anything. But soon, the holiday season arrived and Carolyn became busy, distracted by family and friends gathered at our home for Thanksgiving and Christmas. Our family tradition was for Carolyn's folks to buy all of the groceries and for her mother and her to cook the holiday feast. Carolyn and I loved continuing to entertain, along with the family tradition, and looked forward to these special dinners. And I was looking forward to the leftovers.

But fast forward to our new house. We were settling in and enjoying our new home. At the time, Carolyn's oldest son, Rick, was having marital problems and moved back home. He agreed to finish the basement in lieu of rent, but with the holidays approaching, he ran out of time. Circumstances being what they were, we hired a couple of his friends and the job was completed before the holiday entertaining started. The guys were virtually carrying the tools to the garage as some of Carolyn's friends were coming in the front door to attend a quilt party just before Thanksgiving. This was a gathering of the wives in the new neighborhood.

After the holidays we started to settle down for winter in Minnesota. One day, just after the first of the year, we received a letter from social security that her disability status was to be reviewed by a judge. We didn't know what to do next. We thought we should maybe contact the attorney again or talk to the disability insurer. The process took us a couple of days to work through.

While we pondered what to do next, something out of the blue occurred. A second letter arrived by mail stating the status issue had been resolved. It said payments would start the third Wednesday of the following month, but the back paycheck would be mailed out shortly. It also stated that if we had a problem with this decision we were free to challenge the court's decision. Were they kidding? After all the uncertainty over the last couple of months, we were just relieved the issues were resolved. Challenging the decision was the last thing we thought about.

Why did we receive this blessing? We heard that the Social Security Administration never grants disability like that. We thought that perhaps this is what Dr. Stein meant when he said he would take care of everything. We have since talked to many people and no one has ever seen this happen before or since. We don't really know what happened behind the scenes, but to everyone's amazement, it was taken care of.

Well, the blessing was not without its downside. Social security was not as much money as we had been used to making and we were going to have to learn how to live on less. Carolyn felt bad her 401K would provide little security in the future because her contributions stopped with the rollover to an IRA. However, we did learn how to live on less. With reduced mileage without the commute, Carolyn's car insurance rates went down. We saved in other ways, too, by not eating out as often and doing things for ourselves instead of hiring help.

Sometimes blessings seemed to abound. We were going to have grandchildren living just down the block from our new home. Carolyn's daughter and her husband were expecting and now Carolyn would have the time to spend with this grandchild. We had six other grandchildren already, but we had never had them only a block away. Now we could be active participants in their lives.

As the grandchildren grew up (Cayla was followed by Tyler two years later), Carolyn could baby-sit and get them off to school in the morning. She would usually be there when they got home from school, something that we had not been able to do with the older grandkids. We considered this a double blessing.

Carolyn was quite happy as now she was able to work on her quilting, crafts, and painting. She was elected president of the United Methodist Women's (UMW) group at church. And, as the grandchildren came along, she was able to spend more time with

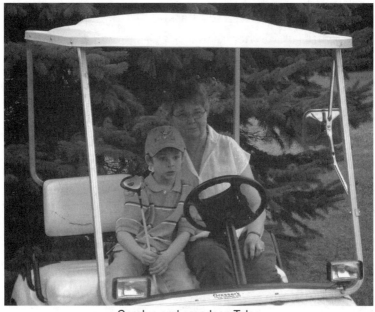

Carolyn and grandson Tyler.

them. All too soon they were going off to daycare and pre-school, so Carolyn gained more free time.

With the access to the golf course Carolyn learned to play golf, and actually got quite good. With her handicap she is able to beat me consistently, even to this day. We also got to spend more time outside in the fresh air and loved spending quality time together. I was still working and away from home from nine hours to eleven hours a day. Carolyn joined the Women's League and played golf every Tuesday for a couple of years. Her girlfriends always took care to see she was partnered up with someone who would look out for her. In the off-season, most of these same girls and their husbands were in our Friday night, once a month, five hundred card club.

Carolyn watched her life continue to change. She remembers, "I used to do a lot of quilting both with friends and with my granddaughter, Jessica. I would go off on quilting weekends with friends. But I got to the point where it got to be too hard just to sew and cut the small squares of material."

Carolyn continued to hold quilting classes for her girlfriends in the neighborhood on Saturday mornings in our basement. She did this as long as she could. But this too came to an end about the time she realized she just couldn't do it all. She struggled to have enough energy left to teach the class for the next Saturday morning.

As for me, Carolyn's son-in-law, Scott, was my men's golf league partner. In the first three years we took two third place finishes and took second place that third year. I think from the very beginning Scott also knew that it was important that the caregiver get some time away.

One day I called home to see how Carolyn was doing, as I often did. The phone rang a long time. When she finally answered it, she gave me some kind of weird story that I had a hard time believing. When I called back to see what was really going on, I was told by my stepson that the ambulance had been there and had taken her to the hospital. She had fallen when trying to answer my call, but said nothing because she didn't want to alarm me.

Carolyn told me what happened as we waited in the emergency room. "I got up to answer the phone; my body didn't move with me and down I went. My ankle was hanging to one side. The pain was awful, but I didn't want to scare Cayla and Tyler whom I was babysitting at the time. So, I did my best to sit up and got the kids to sing songs. We sat there and sang songs until Rick came home. He called the hospital and they sent out the ambulance."

The X-rays revealed she had broken her ankle, not just one break, but three—one break on each of the three major bones in her ankle. It took a number of screws, a wire and titanium plate the size of a credit card to put her back together. After a couple of months she was able to get around again by herself. We suspect that her fall (just like the one she experienced that Saturday morning many years ago), was caused by the Parkinson's symptom called "frozen foot."

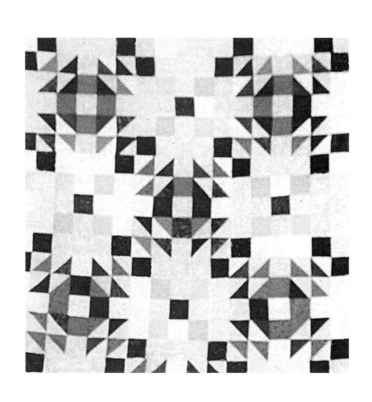

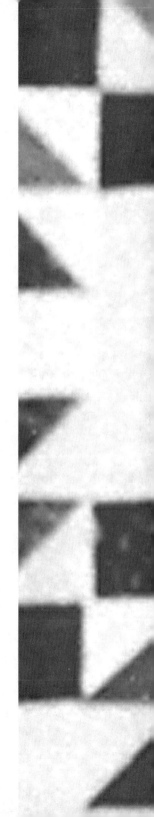

Chapter Three

3

New Options,
New Risks

Life goes on. Carolyn mended quickly and we didn't slow down thanks to vacationing, entertaining and visiting friends and family. Work kept me busy, and babysitting and crafting kept Carolyn occupied. Over the years we had been to Branson, Missouri, and we bought a timeshare condo at the Surry Vacation Resort. A couple of years later we went down to use the condo again thinking we would sell it. By now, Carolyn was having a hard time riding in the car for the thirteen hours it took to get there. When we attended the sales presentation, we didn't sell at all. We traded up for the same unit at Grand Crown Surry Resort on the Thousand Hills Golf Course.

Carolyn continued to quilt. She expanded her quilting so that she was able to create an entire quilt with a new machine she purchased. She wasn't painting much any more, however, as the tremor was affecting her ability to make smooth strokes with a paintbrush.

By 2003 I took off time from work to accompany Carolyn to her doctor appointments because Dr. Stein worked out of the Struthers Parkinson's Center in Golden Valley, Minnesota, a difficult place to drive to as it included an intersection that seemed to be forever under construction. Carolyn just hated that drive. She

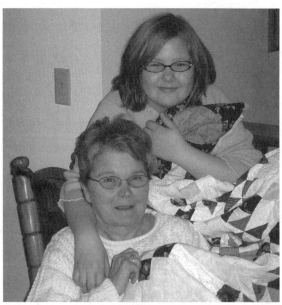
Carolyn and granddaughter Jessica.

never liked driving on the interstate anyway and now she was forced to drive through some of the Twin Cities' worst freeways. For me, it just worked out better to take a couple of hours off work when she had appointments. The company I worked for was fairly understanding about this and allowed me to make up the time during the rest of the week. I didn't have to waste vacation time for these visits, so I was thankful for that.

By now, Carolyn had some sense of what made a good doctor, particularly a good neurologist. She knew her doctors were good ones. A good doctor takes the time to listen to you. They answer your questions, and if you are asked to try a new drug, they will see you get some free samples before purchasing your first prescription. Because of the expense of the medications, when you were at the point Carolyn was at, free samples were a real blessing.

About this time Carolyn discovered there was a nearby Parkinson's specialist, a new doctor who worked out of the Noran Clinic in our old neighborhood. This clinic was just a couple of blocks from our former doctor's clinic and only a couple of minutes from where Carolyn formerly worked. The new doctor, Dr. Shelly Svoboda, was contacted and agreed to take Carolyn's case. Dr. Stein was contacted and he forwarded her records to Dr. Svoboda. Carolyn felt very fortunate that she was able to find a good doctor closer to home. That, and the fact that Dr. Shelly Svoboda was a female, was a bonus blessing in Carolyn's mind.

CAROLYN'S JOURNEY

At their first meeting they hit it off like old friends. After the initial examination Dr. Svoboda suggested that Carolyn think about a new surgical procedure that implanted a device, a device made by a local medical manufacturer, Medtronic, Inc. This was her first introduction to the Activa system.

The Activa surgical implant is an electronic device that works in conjunction with Deep Brain Stimulation (DBS) when micro-electrodes are placed in a critical portion of the patient's brain. The adjustable voltage and frequency aids the patient in controlling symptoms of Parkinson's disease.

Carolyn said, "I will never forget that day. It's a rare opportunity when a doctor like Dr. Svoboda accepts you and you get an appointment. If you turn it down, it may take you another month or more to get another chance to get in to see them. The appointment was set in stone, but then my brother Edwin died. It ended up that I had the first appointment in the morning and that afternoon we attended the memorial service for Ed. It was a very busy day."

When Dr. Svoboda suggested Carolyn think about the surgery, she wasn't quite all together due to the death of her brother. She had been very close to her younger brother Edwin, and he had fought the good fight since the age of nineteen. He had finally lost his lifelong battle with type one diabetes. He was only fifty-three years old, way too young to die. Carolyn felt a little bit better about the end of Ed's life because she and his daughters were at his bedside when the time came for the Lord to take him home. For the last couple of years Edwin lived only a few miles from our house, near Little Elk Lake. The two of them talked on the phone on almost a daily basis. While she would really miss him, I think some of his strength and determination rubbed off on her as she began to process the possibility of having the surgery.

Dr. Svoboda suggested that Carolyn think about what the surgery could mean for her and her quality of life. When we returned home from Edwin's memorial service we went on the Internet and looked up Medtronic's Activa Therapy website. It had some interesting stories and we printed them out so Carolyn could refer to them as she considered her options.

Medtronic Neurological sent us a packet that gave us still more to think about. Part of the information in this packet was a video that showed the condition of patients before and after the surgery and it showed both surgeries, implanting the DBS electrodes and implanting the neurostimulator(s). The video showed how the same patients improved following the surgeries. In one story a man had to crawl just to get around before Activa, and after Activa he could walk. Another man wanted to bowl again, but he couldn't even walk from the house to his car in the driveway. After Activa the man is shown bowling a strike. It said that not all results would be the same and there were risks. At the end of the video it explained all of the risks of surgery, including intercranial hemorrhage, infection and problems with the leads (leads are thin tubes that contain the electrodes) including poor position, migration, dislodgement and breakage.

The Deep Brain Stimulation procedure was described to us as implanting two leads containing the electrodes through the skull into that portion of the brain that was missing the nerve cells that control movement, what we have previously referred to as the "black substance." At that spot the electrical impulses were more like the middle of a thunderstorm in the degenerative condition. With the correct programming of the electrodes, the storm going on in the patient's brain could be calmed and life could become more comfortable for the patient once again.

The patient would go through the first procedure with only a local anesthetic, which means that the patient would be totally conscious throughout the entire seven hour surgery. The brain does not feel pain so the patient can remain awake and will not feel what is going on. However, so that the patient's head does not move during the surgery, it is immobilized in a halo-like frame that is attached to the operating table. Remaining in this frame for several hours can be very uncomfortable for the patient.

Doing the procedure under local anesthesia is preferred because the patient's participation can lead to a better outcome. The patient is asked by the surgical team for input when they place the electrodes and test for results. They might have the patient try to touch their thumb and middle finger together, for example. When the electrodes are in the correct position and activated, the tremor simply goes away. The procedure can be done under general anesthesia, but then the surgical teams may not be sure until later if they got the electrodes in the right place. A correction may need to be done in post-operative surgery.

Carolyn remembers, "When I thought about it, it scared me. When I would get scared, I'd cry about it and then I would pray and we would talk. Then I would cry and pray about it some more. The one thing that kept coming back during every point of consideration was I knew that I could still back out at any time if I wanted to. In the end it turned out to be a quality of life issue. There was the possibility that the tremor could be eliminated, the muscle cramping relieved, and the impairment of voluntary movements eased to a point where I could live a nearly normal life."

After much consideration, Carolyn made the choice to proceed. She started the process by talking with Dr. Svoboda about having the surgery, reading the information from Medtronic, and watching the video again. Once the decision was made, Dr. Svoboda told Carolyn she would be turning her over to the team of doctors at the University of Minnesota Fairview Hospital who would evaluate her and see if she would be a good candidate for the surgery. If she passed the evaluation,, she would remain under their care until such time they released her to come back to Dr. Svoboda who would be her management physician.

Carolyn was more than a little disappointed that after just finding Dr. Svoboda, she was now going to

CAROLYN'S JOURNEY

lose her and have to adjust to a new team of doctors. All that aside, she was still determined to explore having the surgery. This gives you a glimpse of the kind of determination she had in common with her brother, Edwin. She was ready for the future and whatever lay ahead. Carolyn continued to show this iron will and positive attitude that was her driving force to a nearly normal life.

Another factor that arose while contemplating the surgical alternative was the cost of the maintenance drugs Carolyn was taking at this time. She had to medicate up to eight times a day, with the cost of her medications running about eight hundred dollars per month. While we managed the cost using my health insurance drug coverage, it was running our credit card bills through the roof. Her symptoms were also getting worse as the tremor was almost constantly evident. On her left side the tremor never ceased. She described the muscle cramps in her legs as if the muscles were trying to rip her legs apart from the middle. This was never more evident than when she rode in the car.

Three of our five kids lived in the north and northeast suburbs of Minneapolis, in Camden, Spring Lake Park, and Blaine. All are a commute from our home of about thirty-five minutes to an hour, depending on traffic. By the time we would arrive at their homes she was in so much pain that it was almost unbearable. As previously mentioned, we owned a condo in Branson, Missouri, which is a thirteen-hour drive from home, and the last time we had been there was in the spring of 2001. She would never have been able to make that ride by the spring of 2003. The pain of the cramping and the tremors continued to worsen.

The other effect of the cramping was she could no longer even sit at her sewing machine or use her quilting machine. All of her normal activities were so painful that her quality of life was deteriorating. In the summer of 2004, as she was about to start the testing process, the pain was so severe she wondered if she would be able to make the commute to the University of Minnesota Fairview Hospital. However, she was determined to persevere regardless of what she had to endure to gain a nearly normal life.

Carolyn recalls, "I used to love my flowers and gardening, but I couldn't get up and down by 2003 to care for my plants. The physical parts of gardening, the parts you don't even think about when you're feeling good, became a barrier and I couldn't do anything around the yard. As I could not help Victor, our yard deteriorated. We had built an English walk-through garden a few years back and Victor was good at keeping it weed-free, but his job prevented him from routine upkeep. The pond would get cloudy so you couldn't even see the goldfish. By the end of every summer the weeds outgrew anything we were trying to grow. The deer that lived in the neighborhood loved us as we kept day lilies that they thought were dessert. The deer were also fond of our cranberry bush. They would visit our yard in the middle of the night for a snack."

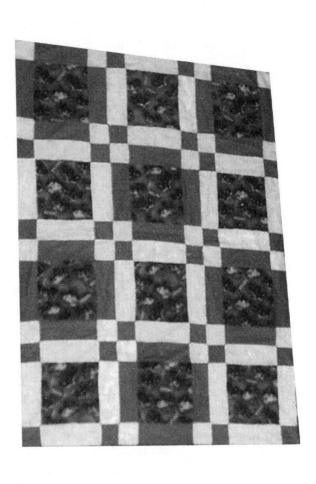

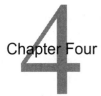

Chapter Four

The Breakthrough

Carolyn was scheduled for evaluation at the University of Minnesota Fairview Hospital as the first step toward the actual surgical procedure. We were told the evaluation, consisting of several tests, would take two days. There would be an interview session where both Carolyn and I would be tested by neurologists and a physiologist. This would take about three hours for Carolyn and about an hour and a half for me. Following the initial testing, Carolyn was then questioned by the team members who would be involved with the approval process. This approval process included almost everyone that would be directly involved in the surgical arena during surgery.

If Carolyn had any reservations about the evaluation process aside from the drive time, she didn't know enough before hand to be nervous about it. The drive to the hospital was during rush hour that first morning and while Carolyn had some discomfort, it wasn't as bad as she had feared. When the questioning started she quickly became nervous as teams of doctors and nurses began asking her question after question. To Carolyn it seemed as if they were asking her questions made up by some kind of crazy person.

For example, she was asked the name of the current president of the United States. When she told them it was George Bush they wanted her to start with him and list previous presidents backwards, for example, Clinton, Bush, and so on. She was asked to spell words correctly and also to spell them backwards. She was feeling dumb and doubted that she would ever qualify for this procedure.

Dr. Mary Sullivan, one of the team members, and I were talking after I finished the testing process. She had some questions about my answers. I mentioned that I did not like the multiple-choice answers to a couple of questions. She told me she also didn't like the limited options to those questions and if she had the time and resources she would like to scrap the test and start over. As this was impossible, this test was the best one currently available, she felt.

By the way, these concerns also included and applied to some of the questions that Carolyn was given as well. The multiple-choice answers for the questions were created by a person whose experience wasn't the same as ours—perhaps a person who never really had Parkinson's—leaving results less than desirable.

As we left for home at the end of the first day of testing Carolyn said to me, "That was the biggest waste of time and money; I'll never get approved for the surgery."

The second round of testing took place the following day. Carolyn didn't look forward to the drive in for the second day any more than the first. She felt bad about how she had done with the tests the first day. With very little hope of passing, along with the pain during the commute she thought, "What is the point?" Again, we made the trip at morning rush hour, increasing her stress, not to mention that the pain was worse that second day. She felt every little bump in the road. In the event she passed the testing, a brain scan would take place at a separate appointment. Luckily for Carolyn, that scan was scheduled directly after the second day of testing.

There was also a final interview with the team surgeon, Dr. Robert Maxwell. This appointment was scheduled separately, and would require yet another trip into the University Hospital to see him at his office.

The second day was more of the same, but this time she was on her own because I had to return to work. I had arranged for our new step-granddaughter to come down and pick Carolyn up after the brain scan. It took a long time for them to find one another, as she wasn't familiar with the University campus area. During the brain scan Carolyn was so tired she fell asleep during the procedure. She was even more convinced after day two that she was not going to be a candidate for the surgery.

However, to her surprise, in a one-on-one meeting with nurse Maggie Bebler, the final decision was that Carolyn was a good candidate and they would schedule her within six months to a year for the surgery. It had not even dawned on Carolyn that when the brain scan had been ordered she had already passed the evaluation.

Carolyn remembers, "The testing was dumb as far as I was concerned, but when I mentioned that to one of the doctors, he was kind enough to explain the logic behind the test questions. He explained that the brain works in different areas depending on what kind of question you are given. So, when they asked about the presidents, that question triggered a different area of the brain than being asked to spell a word, or to spell a word backwards. The doctor then explained the DBS electrodes affected some of these same areas of the brain. The doctors' review of my answers would tell them if the area of the brain was working properly now and whether or not it would be working after the neurostimulator was delivering its electrical charge to that same area."

We had a conversation with nurse Maggie about the nearing fall and winter seasons and how difficult the commute to and from home would be for us from Zimmerman and back. We asked if it was possible to get the procedure done before the bad weather came.

Then, to our surprise, in early July, Carolyn got the call. She was scheduled to have the surgery in two months. This worked out so that Carolyn's first surgery, to implant the electrodes in the brain, would be in mid-September and the second, to implement the neurostimulator near the collarbone, two weeks later, around the first of October. Sometimes it pays to pray about things like this, or maybe it just pays to talk to Maggie. However, Carolyn was now quite sure that God was indeed watching over her.

One thing that Carolyn had been told was to keep her expectations realistic. We later learned that Medtronic encourages doctors to tell their patients to have realistic expectations because if a patients' expectations are unrealistic, they may think the procedure was unsuccessful. We agree with keeping expectations realistic. The benefits for Carolyn have been outstanding, but not everyone will walk away from the surgery with the same results.

The following are a few helpful guidelines, put together by Doctors Okun & Foote, of what to expect from Deep Brain Stimulation.

University of Florida Mnemonic Device for Patients With Parkinson's disease Considering DBS:

*D*oes not cure.

*B*ilateral DBS is often required to improve gait, although sometimes unilateral DBS has a marked effect on walking.

*S*mooths out the on/off fluctuations.

*I*mproves tremor, bradykinesia (slowness), stiffness (rigidity), and dyskinesia in most cases, but may not completely eliminate them.

*N*ever improves symptoms that are unresponsive to your best "on." For example, if gait or balance do not improve with best medication response, it is very unlikely to improve with surgery.

*P*rogramming visits are likely to occur many times during the first 6 months, and then follow-up visits as frequently as every 6 months. There will be multiple adjustments in the stimulator and in the medications.

*D*ecreases medications in many, but not all patients.

Our appointment with the surgeon, Dr. Maxwell, was messed up somewhere along the line. When we arrived for Carolyn's appointment, Dr. Maxwell was just about to leave for another meeting across town. Dr. Maxwell said he would not charge us for the office visit, but stayed with us for about twenty more minutes. He tried in that amount of time to walk Carolyn through what was to happen in both of the surgeries. This included the staging of the two sessions, admission the morning of the first surgery, the halo stereo tactic frame fit, and the DBS placement. He also discussed the MRI/ CT scanning, as well as the incisions to be made in the scalp, at the side of the head, at the ear, and so forth. We knew from the Medtronic video what Dr. Maxwell was talking about as it shows the patient's involvement during the electrode placement. Subsequent testing was also discussed, and after our conversation we thought we had all the facts we needed.

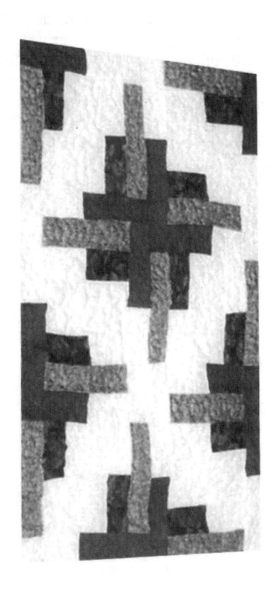

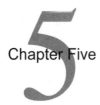

Chapter Five

The First Surgery

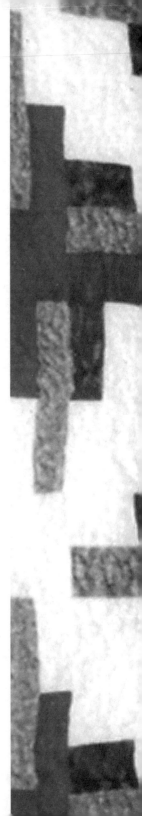

The day of the surgery finally arrived. We left the house a little after 3:00 AM in order to be at the hospital on the University of Minnesota campus by 5:30 AM. Carolyn was excited that the day had finally arrived. She felt a little trepidation on the drive in, but that kept her mind off the fact that her leg muscles felt like they were tearing themselves apart from the kneecap in both directions.

We met Carolyn's son, Jim, and his wife Melissa at the hospital sign-in area, as well as Carolyn's brother, Dan, and her sister-in-law, Mary. We were in the prep area when our minister, Pastor Dan Hair, arrived. We took time for a short devotional, then Carolyn was off to be fitted with the halo.

Carolyn was reminded that she could be put under or stay awake throughout surgery; she had elected to stay awake. The information from the video, what she learned during the evaluation, and Dr. Maxwell's advice that a better outcome could be expected if she remained awake, had convinced her that it was in her own best interest to be a participant in the placement of the electrodes in her brain.

The process begins by shaving off hair in the area where the medical devices will be implanted on the head. We had been warned that there were two nurses who did the head shaving; one liked to shave off all of your hair and the other would take just the hair from around the specific areas that the surgeon required. Carolyn lucked out and had just the partial head-shave.

The halo, which is a square titanium head frame that allows the surgeon to be extremely accurate when implanting the probes in the brain, was then installed. The first attempt was not successful—the halo felt uncomfortable. So before Carolyn actually went into surgery, she was sent back to have the halo removed and repositioned so that it was a little more comfortable.

Carolyn recalls, "All this time the doctors and the nurses kept talking to me. They don't want you to fall asleep. When we arrived in the operating room I looked around at all of the people who were there. The doctors, the nurses, and even an "angel" from Medtronic, Kathleen Lynch, was there to oversee the operation." (Carolyn didn't know who Kathleen was at the time of the surgery, but she would be showing up in our lives more than just this once, in the future.)

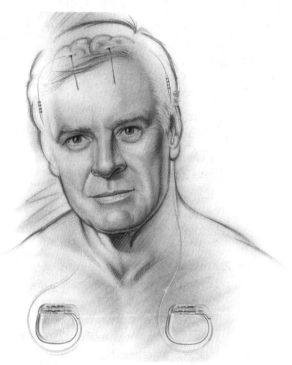

Two holes are drilled in the skull during the first surgery. The two neuro-stimulators are implanted in the chest area during the second surgery. Illustration reprinted with the permission of Medtronic, Inc. © 2002

"During the actual surgery there was little pain," says Carolyn. "The drilling process produced a little pressure. (Two holes about the size of a dime are drilled through the skull.) You know what is going on, but you don't really care. At least I didn't. They were always talking to me and I could hear the drill. About six hours into the surgery I had the feeling that my head weighed about a hundred pounds."

It was about this time that Carolyn heard them talking to one another about a fishing trip that Doctor Maxwell had just returned from. Carolyn shouted to the whole surgical theater, "Will you finish that story and get on with this operation? I want to get this thing off of my head."

Doctor Maxwell came over and patiently explained that they were waiting for the MRI/CT scan to show them that the first electrode was correctly in position and it would be just a little longer. She looked around and could see all of the computer screens showing the MRI/CT scanning progression. She then understood what the wait was all about.

Back in the waiting room, a woman on the phone kept us informed regarding the series of events as each phase was completed. She explained that it had taken about an hour for the original installation of the halo, and that the halo was so uncomfortable for Carolyn that it would have to be taken off and reinstalled a second time, taking another hour. It would also take about four hours to insert the first probe that would place the electrodes, then a pause for the MRI/CT scan, and about forty-five minutes to insert the second probe that would place the second set of electrodes. I'm sure that the voice told me who she was, maybe even a couple of times, but I was under stress at this point and I really don't remember her name.

Carolyn related later that she didn't remember much after the pause for the MRI/CT scan until she was in the recovery room. She woke up for a few minutes to see the family members in the recovery room. She would tell us later, "I was happy that you were there for me. But, really, all I wanted to do was to sleep. I also remember that I silently took time for a little thank you prayer to God for

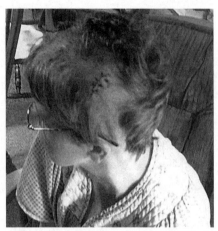

Stitches show spot where one of the leads was implanted in Carolyn's skull.

being there for me during the surgery and for guiding everyone involved through it."

She awoke sometime during evening visiting hours to find her son, Rick, and his wife Kristy, there to visit. After they left, she fell back to sleep. She awoke once more during the evening to find Dr. Tuite checking her incisions. He asked her not to pick at the scabs on her head. From then on, she slept through the night.

Carolyn's daughter, Carla, and grandson, Tyler, came down to the hospital to pick her up after this first phase of the surgery. While her ride home was not pleasant, she managed to endure the entire sixty miles.

She had friends and family to stay with her while she recovered. Her good friend, Penny, was there every day. Some days Penny would be relieved by our daughter-in-law, Melissa, who drove from Blaine in the morning after getting her children off to school.

While recovering, Carolyn realized how many get-well cards and gifts she had received. She felt so special that she was included on the prayer chain, not only at our church, but at a number of local churches, plus at least two churches in California, where both her Aunt Shirley, along with Uncle Earl & Aunt Audrey, lived. She felt blessed so many people cared about her enough to do these nice things for her. Blessings were beginning to take on a new meaning for her.

Carolyn's daughter, Carla, who lived just down the street, would also stop in every night on her way home from work and check on her mom. She would stop with the grandchildren so that they could give Grandma hugs and kisses, even if Grandma looked a little scary.

One problem arose the first week home from the surgery because of how Carolyn kept track of her medications. She kept them all in one bowl and she always seemed to know which ones she had to take and when, even though she didn't write anything down.

While she was still on multiple medications, which she was taking several times each day, her system failed her—she managed to get herself higher than a kite. Her daughter Carla got to the house before I got home from work that particular day and found Carolyn in a confused state of mind. The more Carla tried to reason with her the more Carolyn would giggle.

Carla was a little put out that no one knew what was going on with Carolyn's drugs. She called the local pharmacy and with their help identified all of the pills in the bowl. She also found some pills that Carolyn wasn't supposed to be taking at all. That accounted for the silly state of mind that she had found her in. Carla solved the problem with a daily pill dispenser, putting together the pills prescribed each day for a specific time.

Our advice from this experience, whether you put your drugs in a bowl or use another system, is to make sure other people know when you're supposed to take your medications and what the exact dose should be. Carolyn was only silly and high, but it could have been worse; she could have overdosed as well as not.

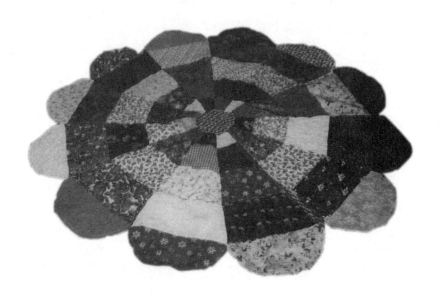

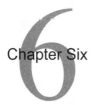

Chapter Six

The Second Surgery

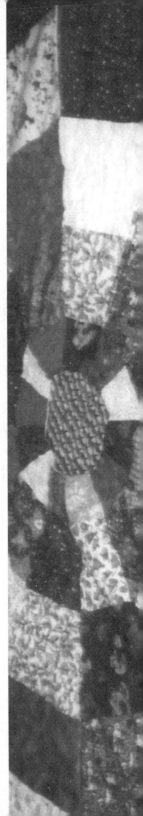

Ten days later, the second surgery was scheduled for about two o'clock in the afternoon. Dr. Maxwell scheduled his surgery days in two parts, doing the first half of the surgery early in the morning and scheduling the generator implants in the afternoon. At the time of the second surgery, nothing was turned on yet, so Carolyn still suffered from the muscle cramping and the tremor. As far as she was concerned, this surgery and activation of the electrodes could not happen quickly enough.

Carolyn was put under for the implant surgery, which only took about an hour and a half. This was a "quick" surgery compared to the six to eight hours for the installation of the deep brain stimulation electrodes. Because she was not conscious during this second operation, Carolyn has no memory of what went on. All she knew was when she came to, she hurt again. All she really wanted to do was sleep.

This is what happened while she was under sedation. Dr. Maxwell connected the cabling to the leads that contained the electrodes. Then he routed the cabling under the skin from the top of the skull to the neck, and then down to the chest cavity where the neurostimulator is placed. Carolyn's neurostimulator is in a crevasse between her shoulder and her rib cage on the left-hand side of her upper chest.

Carolyn spent the night in the hospital after the neurostimulator implant surgery. I had visited Carolyn after work the night after surgery, but because of my job, I had to be at work while she underwent the neurostimulator surgery. Before leaving the hospital the next day, nurse Maggie came up to the room for the initial programming and settings to the device which would remove the muscle cramping and tremor.

My employer was not being very cooperative about my having additional time off if it interfered with the company's schedule. To be honest about the situation at work, the company was simply reacting to a situation that I had been warned about by the doctors. They told me that the caregiver will be affected by the stress and it could cause memory lapse. Now I can say, looking back, that I was not performing to my usual level of productivity. I was not about to admit to anyone that worrying about her was the cause of memory lapses and concentration problems. Later, I found that not admitting to this would eventually cost me my job.

Carolyn does not have very fond memories about the trip home the next day. The ride home was horrific as she again felt every little bump in the road. Her brother and sister-in-law, Dan and Mary, who came down to pick her up and bring her home, owned a sport utility vehicle. The short wheel base vehicle with stiff suspension had a rougher ride than she was used to and so, by the time she arrived home, she had endured about as long a ride as she could take. But again she had survived the sixty-mile trip.

She remembered later, "It felt as though I had a little person inside my head with a big hammer drumming away and I was so glad to get out of that car. At first, I thought I was going to die, and then I was afraid that I wouldn't. I recalled that I had really wanted to die until I arrived home and got into bed." Dan and Mary had stayed waiting for me to get home from work and were talking in the living room when I arrived.

Carolyn would recall that until she drifted off to sleep she wanted to tell them, "Just let me die." Then she remembered how hard it had been to lose their younger brother just a few months earlier. Dan had also lost his first wife some years earlier, and this reminded her of something that her brother Ed had said to her. He told her, "Your time on earth was not yet done because the family needs you." She remembered she had promised Ed that she would watch over his two daughters and his grandchildren. She closed her eyes and prayed that the good Lord would help her through this. She believed that her prayers were answered. It seemed as though Jesus said to her in her sleep, "In time, this too will pass."

Carolyn slept a lot when she got home from surgery and she was so happy for the caregivers, Penny Rice, Melissa, and myself, who took care of her during this phase of the recovery. Penny recalls the following about the surgery and recovery. "Carolyn came out of it very well, but naturally, with pain and also some amount of confusion. Considering the major surgery she had just had, this was to be expected. I spent several days with her, making sure she had her meals, took naps and so forth. Prior to the surgery Carolyn had quite a severe tremor affecting her head and arms. We were amazed that she had no sign of those prior symptoms following the surgery. By the time a few days had passed, she seemed so much better and still no sign of tremors. Her medications were also cut way down. Before surgery she was on many medications and after the surgery she was down to only one or two and only a couple times a day."

The days turned into weeks, and Carolyn returned to the university for tweaking on the programming of the device and for check-ups from both nurse Maggie and Dr. Maxwell.

Carolyn's first appointment after the surgery was with Dr. Maxwell. He found her stitches were healing properly and there was no evidence of cable migration (moving where it shouldn't be moving). He then turned her over to nurse Maggie, who made some minor programming changes. The device has a number of different options. The individual electrodes

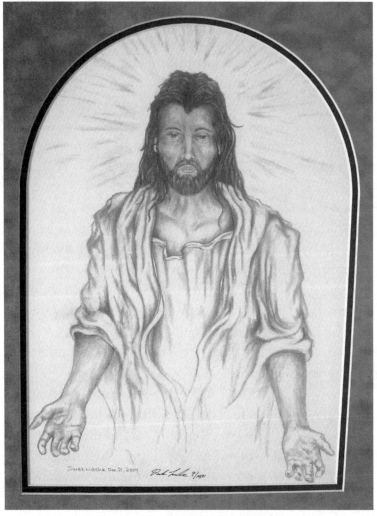

"In time, this too will pass" (sketch by Derek Lusche).

can be programmed to their own specific frequency and voltage as well as the side of the patient's body that they are aimed to affect the most. The original programming after the second surgery was so close to perfect that the only thing changed on this first appointment was a slight increase in voltage to 1.5 volts.

During our second appointment for programming tweaking, we were waiting for Maggie in the reception area. Maggie arrived and took us into the examining room. Maggie thought that she should increase the voltage as Carolyn was showing signs of weakness and lack of energy. She increased the voltage from 1.5 volts to 1.8. After she did so, Maggie remembered that she had a stash of Stalevo, the drug Dr. Svoboda had prescribed for Carolyn, so she excused herself and ran upstairs to retrieve these samples. Carolyn and I were left in the examination room. About two minutes after Maggie left, Carolyn started to complain of the higher voltage making her very anxious. By the time that Maggie returned, Carolyn was flopping around on the examination bed like a fresh-caught fish in the bottom of a boat. Maggie turned her back down to 1.6 volts and apologized for the error, but Carolyn soon felt she was better than ever.

Soon it came time to be turned back over to Dr. Svoboda. After this second meeting with Dr. Maxwell and nurse Maggie, we thought our relationship was over with the University Fairview Hospital at this time. Later we would find out we still needed to go back every six months. The hospital could still track her programming even if Dr. Svoboda was doing the programming at this point.

One day Carolyn got a call from a person that had talked to nurse Maggie. Maggie had told this patient that if they had any questions about the surgery to call Carolyn and ask her about her experience. Carolyn was slowly becoming an Activa ambassador, and Maggie wasn't shy about sending people to talk to Carolyn.

Carolyn tried to be as honest as she could about the reality of having this surgery. She would list problems she had while going through the evaluation process, the problems with the halo device, and the challenges on the day of the first surgery. Sometimes she told the story about Dr. Maxwell's fishing trip. In the end she would tell everyone, "None of that matters; I would go back and do this whole thing all over again tomorrow to attain a nearly normal life."

We discovered that because Medicare approves this operation, the largest portion is covered by the plan. Our supplemental AARP insurance covered nearly all of the rest of the expense. If a patient is as lucky as Carolyn, his or her drug cost can be greatly reduced after surgery if programming has stabilized the symptoms.

It was also about this time that everyone we met told us how inspiring Carolyn's journey was, and that's when we decided to sit down and write this book. This would enable us to, hopefully, help others to understand Parkinson's and the benefits that Carolyn has derived from Activa therapy.

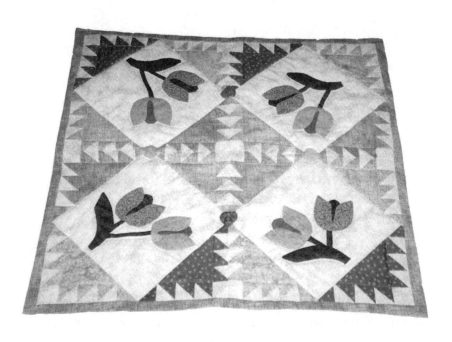

7
Chapter Seven

The Ambassadorship

Six months after the surgery we received a phone call from the education department of Medtronic Neurological. They asked if Carolyn would come to the Le Meridien, a Minneapolis hotel, to be a volunteer at a Parkinson's seminar for Dr. Svoboda. A doctor from New York City was going to be teaching a section of the seminar, along with Dr. Svoboda, on programming the device. The caller advised that Carolyn would be reimbursed for her time. The seminar fit perfectly into our schedule as we were just preparing for a vacation cruise to the

Mexican Riviera and a California road trip to see some of Carolyn's relatives. The seminar would take place the Sunday after we returned from vacation.

Carolyn didn't have to think twice. She had thought about all of the things she could do to help people with Parkinson's and she was ready to do it. She also thought of all she could do with a little extra spending money and said that she would be happy to participate.

Our vacation cruise of the Mexican Riviera started by flying to San Diego to meet the ship, and my cousin, Al, and his wife, Sue. They picked us up at the airport and took us to our hotel. We checked in, went up to our rooms, and returned to the lobby where we met my son, Mike, and his wife, Dena. The six of us went out for dinner at Fleming's in downtown San Diego and had a great time.

The following morning after breakfast, the four of us headed to the pier to get aboard our cruise ship and enjoy the first leg of our vacation. The first two days were at sea sailing to Ixtapa-Zihuatanejo, where we took a scenic shopping tour.

The next stop was Acapulco, where one of the highlights for me was a stop to see the cliff divers. The cliff divers are family members from six families who have been jumping off these cliffs now for several generations. They jump from two heights, one being about twenty feet. That may not sound like any big deal, but the sea below is only six feet deep. Over the years a couple of the divers have been hurt, but they dive seven days a week all year round. The first time that I remember seeing the divers was in Elvis Presley's movie "Fun in Acapulco" back in the 1960s. I asked if that movie had increased tourism and our guide said that it did, for about two weeks. The guide also said that Elvis made his next six movies in Hawaii.

The natives at every stop on these tours were trying to sell souvenirs to everyone on each bus who arrived to see the divers. When Carolyn told one old lady that she didn't want the plate she was selling, the crazy woman hit Carolyn in the leg with the plate she was trying to sell her. Carolyn said that it hurt at the time, but we both thought the pain would go away in a little while. We finished our tour and boarded the ship for Manzanillo. We continued our tour. Getting on and off the ship was no problem for Carolyn.

We returned to San Diego. Al went back to the hotel and got their truck. He picked us up across the street from the ship and brought us to the car rental building. Then Al and Sue left to go back to Arizona. They still wanted to finish their winter vacationing. Carolyn and I picked up a Dodge Stratus four-door and headed for Fresno, California, where her Aunt Shirley lived as well as a number of other cousins and their families.

The first night we stayed at her aunt Shirley's house, Carolyn got up to go to the bathroom in the middle of the night and she tripped, just as she had on that Saturday morning so long ago. This time her fall landed her on her side, right on top of Shirley's sewing machine cabinet. Activa therapy didn't fix everything, or so it seemed.

By morning Carolyn woke up ill with black and blue marks all the way down her side. She had diarrhea and complained of all of her old symptoms. We discussed taking her to a local hospital. She started having tremors and her face was really showing the dyskinesia, just like before her surgery. I retrieved a hand-held remote to check the status mode of the device. I had only been shown how it operated once before. I checked and it appeared that her implant was off. So, to be absolutely sure that it was off, I turned the implant off with the remote. I then turned it back on using the remote.

I called the Noran Clinic back in Minneapolis. The doctor on duty advised us not to take Carolyn to a hospital under any circumstance. He had me turn the device off again and then turn it back on to make sure she was indeed turned on. He instructed me to give her another dose of her pills, let her rest about an hour, and then call him back. Fifty-five minutes later Carolyn was lying on Shirley's sofa. After shaking for the entire fifty-five minutes, she calmed right down a few minutes later. The tremor was gone, the dyskinesia was no longer noticeable and she said that the muscle cramping was also subsiding.

What we learned from this experience was it took about twenty-four hours before the device being turned off would become evident. We were able to piece together that when we were leaving the ship in San Diego the ship must have had their electronic security screening device on at the ramp to the pier, to prohibit guests walking off with unpaid items. That must have been what turned Carolyn's implant off. By this time, Carolyn was feeling ever so much better, but she was still complaining about the lady that had hit her leg with a plate in Acapulco. We also noticed she started to favor that leg and her walk was starting to be affected.

I was glad that we didn't have to take her to the hospital because the fall made her appear like she had been beaten. Her whole side was black and blue. The bruise extended from her armpit at the top and went down to her waist. To be perfectly honest, the fact that the doctor didn't want us going to the hospital was just fine with me. You know how they ask patients if they feel safe at home when they are admitted to the hospital? I was really afraid that in this case they would not even have bothered with the question. They would have just called the cops. I would have gone straight to jail; I wouldn't get a chance to pass go or to collect two hundred dollars had we taken her to the hospital.

Later that day we got together with relatives and had some good times. Carolyn's other aunt, Bertha, was there from the nursing home where she lived. She hadn't seen Carolyn since we were there in 1994 for Shirley's fiftieth wedding anniversary. This get-together was a family reunion to remember and we took lots of photos.

The next day one of Shirley's grandchildren, who worked at the local Chevrolet dealership, took us to a party they were throwing for the employees and their guests. We felt right at home because my cousin, Al, had just sold his Chevrolet dealership after over thirty years of selling me new Chevrolets.

The next morning we were off to the coast to see Carolyn's Uncle Earl and his wife, Audrey. From their place the next day we went to the Hearst mansion, and visited the area north up the coastal highway. Everyone should see the mansion at least once in their lifetime. The sea lions were all over the beach just north of the mansion and an old hippy told us all about them. They are only the females, he told us, and they are all pregnant. They were close to giving birth. The females sleep on the shore. They don't breath; they exhale all of the air from their body and rest and wait to give birth. Somehow they were quite fine just lying there. If you see movement, that is the baby inside moving around.

The following day we took a trip south to Solvag, California, where the movie *Sideways* was filmed. Carolyn is part Danish and she had always heard so much about this Danish town in California. It is a beautiful little town with some of the nicest people you'll ever meet. We even managed to find a Native American casino on the route that Audrey told us to take home. We stopped there to play the slots for a while and had lunch.

Earl and Audrey had a wonderful dinner ready when we arrived back. The next day came quickly and it was time to return to San Diego. So, we headed south to join up again with my son, Mike, and his wife. We stopped to see the Crystal Cathedral along the way. Carolyn loves to watch Dr. Schuller on Sunday mornings before attending church. To see this place and take the tour was very special to her.

The Ambassadorship

We went out to dinner that night with Mike, Dena, and Dena's dad and step mom. This was the first time that Carolyn and I had a chance to meet Dena's dad. We had visited Mike and Dena in 1994, the year after they got married. On that trip they met us in Fresno, but there was no chance to go south and meet her dad.

The next day we were on our way back home, arriving about 11:00 PM at the Minneapolis-St. Paul airport. Carolyn's favorite son-in-law, Scott, met us there and took us home. Boy, it sure was good to get back. We were both looking forward to a good night's sleep in our own bed.

Later, as the bruise from the plate on Carolyn's leg healed, we were told she had altered her walking gait to compensate for the pain she had been feeling. While Medicare wasn't wild about a Parkinson's patient getting physical therapy for gait problems, Dr. Svoboda wouldn't take no for an answer and they gave in. They let Carolyn have two rounds of therapy over the next couple of months. Carolyn slowly adjusted her walk through the physical therapy sessions. She regained her walk and gait and was put on a workout program that she still does sometimes. While our lives are filled with multiple blessings, some events that happen to you are not without consequence.

Carolyn had been thinking about the Medtronic presentation quite a bit the last days of our vacation. She had never been to any event like this and wondered what they would have her do.

That Sunday morning we got up early and drove to downtown Minneapolis, located the hotel, and were greeted by Kathleen Lynch from Medtronic, the woman who was Carolyn's angel in the first surgery. She told us that we were a little early. However, she said we were welcome to observe a woman and her doctor go through the teaching phase that would lead to Carolyn's part in this.

Dr. Svoboda came in and assured Carolyn that the changes in programming would be temporary and should make her feel better. Dr. Svoboda had learned that the doctor from New York who was also part of the demonstration was very good at what he did. She was so impressed, in fact, that she talked about going to New York to learn more about how he works with his patients. They had agreed to set something up after the seminar.

It was soon time for Carolyn to go on. Dr. Svodoba introduced her to the other doctor and doctors in the class. Carolyn had been scheduled last and by this time some of the students had their bags packed and were running to catch a cab to go to the airport. But those who stayed had questions for her and for Dr. Svodoba. The doctors made changes to Carolyn's programming to see the effect it would have on her. She walked through the room to show the students how the programming changed her control, her walk, gait and balance. Now remember, this was only a day after we returned from California, so Carolyn was still suffering with the sore leg. She explained the incident in Acapulco to make sure they didn't confuse the pain problem for the walking problems of Parkinson's.

Carolyn was through and we made our way to a luncheon following the presentation. We met with Maggie at the luncheon and chatted. Maggie was teaching another class in an adjacent conference room. Then we made our way down to the lobby and had our car brought around. On the way home, we talked about how Carolyn felt about doing this again. She wanted to continue to help individuals contemplating the surgery, felt this was very rewarding, and said she would do it again if asked. And they did ask again. She was paid for several appearances and we just showed up at several others to show support for Dr. Svodoba.

Carolyn had written some thoughts about her journey with Parkinson's, which was helpful in preparing this book. We worked in our spare time reading material from every source we could find and located valuable websites. The actor Michael J. Fox was one of her personal heroes as he was so young when he got Parkinson's. When a new magazine showed up with his face on the cover, you knew it was coming home with her from the grocery store.

As I mentioned before, Michael J. Fox's website is very informative. Sometimes having the kind of resources he has isn't an advantage. His surgery had actually burned a portion of the brain so DBS won't work in his brain any more. He still needs help, but until somebody comes up with a system that will work in a brain with the surgery he had, he's stuck with what he has for the time being. We hope some day doctors help him get back to a nearly normal life.

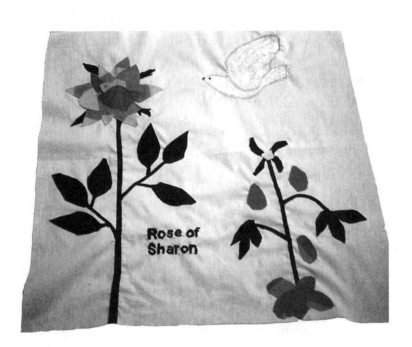

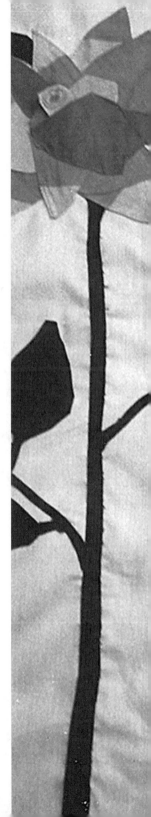

8
Chapter Eight

Blessings With a Nearly Normal Life

Carolyn's day-to-day life after surgery was a change beyond her wildest expectations. It changed her perspective on life. She now experiences more energy than she had in some time. Her spiritual eyes were opened by this journey. Carolyn has gained strength to perform chores around the house she hadn't felt able to do for quite some time. She now works on the gardens around the house. She takes care of the housework, except for the vacuuming. The vacuum seemed to drain her energy when she was starting her day. With the tremor gone and the muscle cramping gone, she feels like people aren't always staring at her due to her disability. She feels people now look at her with a sense of inspiration on how well she has done since surgery.

This happened, we believe, by living through the total experience of the journey. She now has a different outlook on life, a more positive mindset, and sees the everyday things in her life through the lens of her new vision. This allows her to see and appreciate blessings big and small contained within them.

The activities Carolyn views as blessings are combined with the day-to-day activities everyone does. Living where we do, Carolyn plays a round of golf with me every chance she can. She had almost entirely stopped golfing with her girlfriends in the summer of 2005. I hope in the future she will get involved with the women's league or at least with her neighborhood friends.

This past year we tried to address some caregiver issues. Carolyn sometimes has restless nights and she will twitch in her sleep. This muscle twitching often is followed by erratic movements, such as swinging her arms in the air. While I have never been hit by one of these movements, I believe if she ever did connect it might hurt a bit. Sometimes she starts to roll around. This concerns me as she could roll over the edge of the mattress and fall to the floor. That has only happened

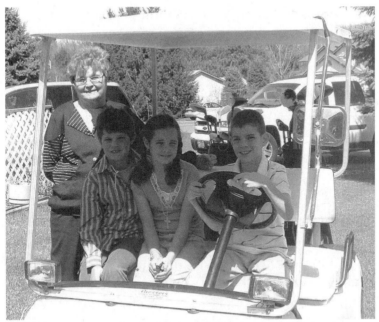

Carolyn with grandkids Nick, Danielle and Luke.

once and she fell softly enough so she didn't harm herself. She has been fortunate in this respect.

At other times she talks in her sleep. This varies from giggling to screaming, and it can scare the life out of me. If it wakes me up in the middle of the night, I can have a hard time getting back to sleep. We asked about this at seminars and have discussed it with Dr. Svoboda. Some of the seminar doctors were sympathetic. Dr. Svoboda said, "If she seems happy, don't worry about it."

While getting a good night's sleep is really important for her, she has said that if I ever feel threatened, then I should go ahead and nudge her and have her roll over.

We were told a change of sleeping position may make the dream go away. We have adopted her suggested strategy and it seems to be working quite well.

Given what we have learned about the drugs, their history and the side effects, I wonder why these symptoms are not more prevalent than they are. We have learned from our support group that maybe people just don't want to talk about them. Also, single people may not have a bed partner or caregiver to tell them what they do while sleeping. Many may wake up in the morning with no recollection of doing anything. Carolyn has never awakened from one of her episodes and remembered her dream, what might have triggered a scream while she was asleep, or what caused her erratic movements.

Our support group meets in Coon Rapids, Minnesota, once a month. We have an excellent co-coordinator who brings us informational guests and entertainment. The meetings don't follow a given agenda, but often include a mix of education and entertainment followed by refreshments. Then we gather in groups with patients at one table and caregivers at another to discuss what we are confronting on a daily basis.

We would like to give a big "thank you" to doctors, like Dr. Svoboda, who take time out of their busy days to join us, answer questions and address the challenges that both patients and caregivers are experiencing. This is invaluable for the patients and the caregivers who truly feel different from other people because of their association with Parkinson's. Sometimes it just helps to talk about situations and know there are others dealing with the same issues.

I would also like to say something about the people who get Parkinson's. I have never met one single person who seemed to feel sorry for himself or herself. To the contrary, both patients and caregivers are usually the first to volunteer if someone needs a helping hand, either in the group or in the community. They are just very nice people who are there for each other if they know that you're having a rough spot in your journey.

We have lived through all of it: the disease progression, the decision to enter into the qualifying process and having the surgery. Having taken this very difficult journey, Carolyn is blessed to have achieved a nearly normal life again. The many blessings that have come our way are not comprehended by others. Prior to living through this experience, we could not have believed our lives would have been touched in this way. While I was working for a living I never thought about myself as an author, but here I am writing this book, telling its inspiring journey, not just for Carolyn, but for everyone with Parkinson's disease.

As Carolyn will tell you, there is another story woven into this journey as well. It is a love story that begins with two teenagers, who remember as if it happened yesterday. They met each other on a 1957 spring morning at one of the first gatherings of a soon-to-be Methodist church in Mounds View, Minnesota. We first met when our folks came to the Sunnyside

Grade School where services were held until the new church was constructed.

That teenage boy and that beautiful girl in the pink dress with all of those crinolines, who for one reason or another went their separate ways, got back together and were married in 1982. They have been on this journey for the majority of the entire time they have been married. They are still in love and committed to each other. And they have dedicated their lives to the best nearly normal life they can bring to each other.

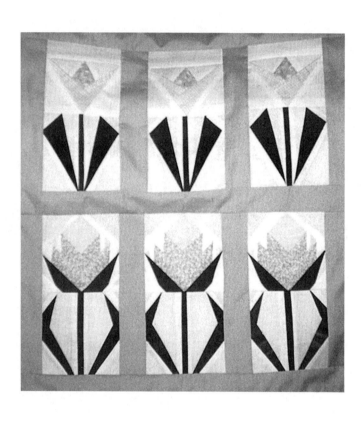

Chapter Nine

The Piano Lessons

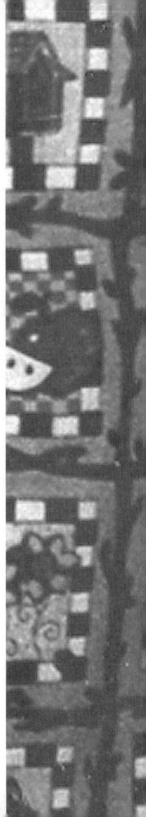

When Carolyn was diagnosed with Parkinson's disease, she gave our piano away to her daughter and son-in-law and the two grandchildren that lived a block away. Her excuse was that our new house didn't have the room for a piano. The truth is that because of the Parkinson's, she hadn't been able to play for some time.

About a year after the first surgery, Carolyn and I decided to make a trip to

Branson to our condo. We were planning to go the first week in December as we had owned our condo for nine years now and had not been there for any Christmas shows. For the last couple of years Carolyn would not have been able to travel that far without experiencing excruciating pain. Since the surgery, it was no problem at all. We started the planning process about the time the grandchildren were heading back to school in the fall of 2005. Our grandson, Tyler, loved the attractions of Branson the last time we were all there as one big family. Tyler was thrilled by every show we went to see.

On our only trip since that vacation, Carolyn and I went alone. While we were there, I won a pair of tickets to the Dutton Family Show. While we were watching the beginning of the show, Sheila, the mom, came out into the audience and picked me to go up and do a number with the band. They got me up on stage and I performed as best I could without any idea what we were going to do. They sang and danced to Elvis's song "All Shook Up" while I played a triangle. They told me to strike it every time the word "love" came up in the song. When they do this, they give the "hapless" performer a copy of the performance on video.

When we returned after that trip we showed everyone the video of me making a fool of myself. From the first time that Tyler saw that video, he wanted to watch it every day when he was babysat by Grandma. During that time the video nearly wore out.

The Piano Lessons

At first it looked like Carolyn's daughter, son-in-law, and Cayla and Tyler would join us for this trip. As much as the grandchildren would have enjoyed going back, their other commitments prevented it. So, we decided to reserve the unit and made plans to finish our Christmas shopping while we were there.

One day in late September our granddaughter, Cayla, out of the blue, asked if grandma Carolyn would teach her to play the piano. Carolyn was taken back but said, "Sure, I'll be happy to show you how to play the piano." After thinking about this for a while she asked her son-in-law, Scott, if he would bring the piano back from their basement. He said, "No problem."

The next weekend we had a dusty old piano in our living room. We knew that after eight years of sitting in

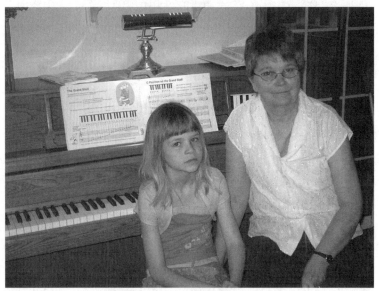

Carolyn and granddaughter Cayla.

their basement that the piano would need to be tuned, so Carolyn set up an appointment for the tuner. Later we had him back a second time to fix a few sticky keys. It soon became apparent that any further repairs done to this old relic were not going to save it. But, all things considered, by the time Thanksgiving approached, the piano was in as good a shape as one could expect from a forty-plus-year-old piano.

In October, Carolyn located a teacher and started to take some piano lessons herself. She thought she had better brush up on her skills before she tried to teach anyone to play. Another little girl in the neighborhood, Holly, also asked if Carolyn would teach her how to play and Holly started taking lessons right away. Carolyn's teacher needed a place to hold a Christmas recital, so Carolyn volunteered and arranged with our church to have the concert held there. Carolyn wasn't so sure that she would even participate.

We made it through Thanksgiving and then we were on our way to Branson. We met my cousin and his wife for breakfast in Owatonna, Minnesota, which turned out to be closer to lunch after driving through the sleet and rain. We had a great time and once again we were off to continue our road trip. The interstate was sleet-covered, very treacherous to drive on, and getting worse. We weren't making very good time from there to Des Moines, Iowa. To make matters worse, I was close to falling asleep at the wheel, and the tension of driving on this sleet-covered roadway was getting to me. We found a gas station, filled the car, and decided to find a room. We found a nice motel and retrieved our bags to stay the night.

We watched the news on TV for a little while and caught up with the world at large. We looked outside to find the weather was clearing and that the restaurant next door was having its parking lot plowed. The snow and sleet had pretty much let up, so we scurried across the parking lot and had supper. The next morning we got into the car and continued down Interstate 35 toward our destination. Stopping only when needed, we made it to the check-in at the condo about four o'clock that afternoon.

Carolyn took this whole week off from practicing her song, "The First Noel" for the recital. She had convinced herself that she would not play in the concert. She was only one of two adults even taking piano lessons from her teacher, and while she never said it out loud, I thought she didn't want to be out-performed by one of those school kids.

In Branson we saw Andy Williams, the Osmonds, the Duttons, and the Gatlins with the "wuniful" Lennon Sisters at the Welk Theater. We wanted to tell the Duttons, who had been so kind to us on our previous visit, how much our grandson had loved that video. I later got a chance to give Sheila and her two daughters a big thank you from Tyler. Branson is a fun town if you like music and live shows. The week flew by and we got all of the shopping done (as well as the gift-wrapping) and were on our way home. We had one light snowfall while we were there, but the locals were still golfing through Tuesday before the snowfall in spite of the nippy weather. On the way home, we were experiencing a rain that we were afraid would turn to ice or snow the farther north we went.

By the time that we made Iowa, with the weather being uncertain, we decided to stay the night. We were back on the road the next morning only to find out that overnight the rain had not frozen on the roads. The farther north we went the rain disappeared and we made it home in good shape. The next couple of days Carolyn put in some really good practices at the piano. She thought that maybe she would participate in the concert after all. Also, her teacher would not take no for an answer.

As the concert was at our church, we were there that night to let people in and helped set up. This kept Carolyn so busy that she had no time to worry about her performance until we sat down to watch the other students play. Carolyn's spot in the concert came a little past the half way mark. It came faster than she had expected and soon she was being introduced.

She sat down and began to play, loving the way the grand piano sounded. She nailed the performance and did it so well that she played the second verse as well. Carolyn got up, took her bow, and came back to her seat, so proud of herself. I had taken the pictures of the students that we knew from our church and the next Sunday gave each of their parents a copy. We were both hits in our own minds. I have to admit I didn't know

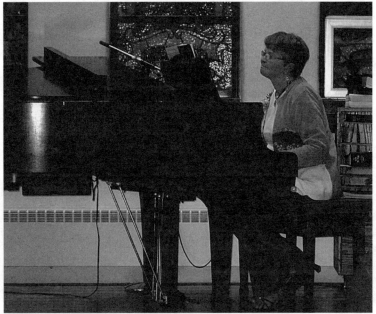
Carolyn playing at the Christmas recital.

if she could pull this off, but as I have stated before, blessings abound when you believe.

You might not think about these little things as blessings while doing them. On reflection, however, the ability to watch the shows in Branson (the professional performers you have admired all of your life) and applying it to Carolyn's recital makes the true meaning of how life is interconnected come to light. I think if Cayla decides to take piano lessons from Grandma Carol, she too will see the whole experience in her life go full circle. And it will bring Cayla closer to the other things that she has learned so far. This could bring about a blessing she wasn't expecting when she asked Grandma to teach her to play the piano.

Carolyn's overall heath since the surgery has been very good. She gets worn out if she tries to do too much and she comes down with a cold now and again, but generally she is in excellent condition and has a nearly normal life. She has been improving her golf game, and she still has her sewing area in the spare bedroom. She has several projects she is doing a little at a time. She practices her piano lessons every day. We gave up on the old piano and replaced it with a much newer one after we returned from Branson. She cooks really great meals, except for grilling. That is my area. We travel, as you have read, and visiting with friends and neighbors is really fun. We even hosted a New Year's Eve party for some of the neighbors recently. So, it seems every day of this nearly normal life is full of new surprises and many, many blessings.

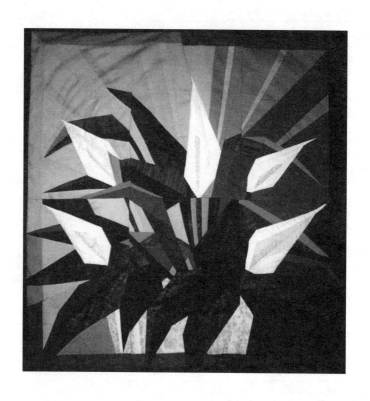

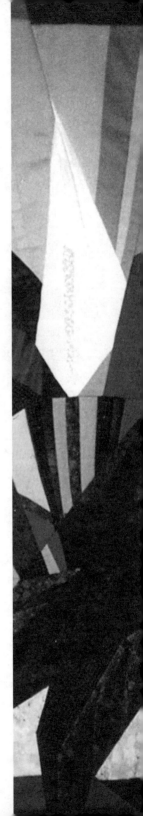

10

Giving Thanks Every Day

Our spiritual life has changed and I believe it is not specifically because of the surgery, or the Parkinson's disease, but because of Carolyn, and in some small way, my own attitude. It's our fight together for a nearly normal life. It is our combined desire to live out whatever comes our way, and keep moving ahead as long as we are able.

We have given you some examples in the previous chapters of how these changes have impacted our spiritual lives through the blessings that it has brought us. In this, the final chapter of this story about Carolyn's journey, we would like to tell you about the sources of some of our blessings. The following is a partial listing of the people who are associated with, or are personally the blessings that we give thanks for every day.

Thank you:

Dr. Shelly Svoboda, for without you, none of this would have happened.

To the neurologist at the Minneapolis Clinic of Neurology and the neurologist from Mayo Clinic for their diagnoses.

Dr. Steven Stein, for your care and guidance through the early years that you were Carolyn's primary Parkinson's physician.

Dr. Paul Tuite, for you and your team, whose vote of confidence enabled Carolyn to become a candidate for the surgery in the first place. That was the inspiration that started us down the road that would lead us to this place in our life and help us back toward a nearly normal life.

Dr. M. Sullivan, for your confidence that Carolyn was of sound mind and a good candidate in the first place.

Dr. Robert Maxwell, for your gifted hands, your talent, and your dedication to the Parkinson's patients in Minnesota and beyond.

For nurse Maggie Bebler, our angel and friend during the process from start to finish.

For Drs. Okun and Foote for letting us use their mnemonic for Parkinson disease patients considering Deep Brain Stimulation.

For all the staff and unsung heroes at University of Minnesota Fairview Hospital, and for that matter, the rest of the Fairview Hospital System, including the physicians and nurses at Northland Regional Hospital, Princeton, Minnesota.

To the staff and doctors of the Noran Clinic for their support.

To our family, Carolyn's:

Daughter, Carla, her husband Scott, my golf partner, and their children, Cayla and Tyler. They are always there for us and are always a blessing in our lives.

Son, Rick, and his wife, Kristy, and their children, Kiel, David, and Jessica. We appreciate their help and support.

Son, Jim, and his wife, Melissa, and their children, Luke, Nick and Danielle, for their assistance with care giving and support when we needed it, even when we didn't recognize it.

Brother, Dan, and his wife, Mary, as they were always ready to drop whatever they were doing and lend a hand to be there for Carolyn.

For her brother, Edwin, who, while he was still here with us, was a spiritual rock from which I believe Carolyn was anchored, such that her belief never varied.

For my family:

Son, Marc, and his wife, Kris, their children old and new, Mitchel, Jaclyn, Erik and Aimee.

Son, Mike, and his wife, Dena, who, though separated by miles, were always in our hearts and we in theirs.

For friends like:

Arvy and Penny Rice, caregivers if needed, and always good friends.

The rest of the community here at Lakeplace Shores who gave us strength at times of need, even if they never realized it.

To our church family at Princeton United Methodist Church, who would step up and carry our load if this journey took us away from our commitment to them.

To my cousin, Al, and his wife, Sue, who have been there for us in times of need and were our occasional travel partners.

To the team that helped us with this book from the beginning, Sandy Olson and Penny Rice, whose proofreading skills kept my text from reading poorly.

From me to my wife, Carolyn, who supplied the inspiration just by living her faith, as well as for the quilts that became a theme. Thank you also for helping me make good choices along the way.

Giving Thanks Every Day

To you, the reader:

Thanks for joining Carolyn and me on this journey. We hope it has been helpful and inspiring for you. You are welcome to contact us at Clictor1@peoplepc.com.

Order Form

Fill out this form (or a photocopy), add the necessary information, and mail it to:

Victor Anderson
28422 133rd St
Zimmerman, MN 55398

Please enclose personal check or money order payable to: Victor Anderson.

You can also order at www.candvbooks.com, email Victor at Clictor1@peoplepc.com, or call him at 763-856-2644.

Author: Victor Anderson
ISBN: 1-930374-23-2

	Cost	Quantity	Total
Carolyn's Journey	$14.95	_____	_____
Numbered lithograph of original charcoal drawing of Jesus by Derek Lusche (p. 69)	$89.95	_____	_____

Subtotal _____

Minnesota residents add 6.5% sales tax ($0.97/bk) _____

Shipping: $3.00 first book, $1.00 each additional book _____

$6.00 for lithograph _____

Total enclosed: _____

Name: _____

Address: _____

City: _____ State: _____ Zip: _____

Phone: (____) _____ Email:_____